Amel DJERBAL
Ahcene SAID OUAMER
Samir TEBANI

Orthopedics MCQs and Case Studies

Amel DJERBAL
Ahcene SAID OUAMER
Samir TEBANI

Orthopedics MCQs and Case Studies

ScienciaScripts

Imprint

Cover image: www.ingimage.com

This book is a translation from the original published under ISBN 978-620-6-70611-3.

Publisher:
Sciencia Scripts
is a trademark of
Dodo Books Indian Ocean Ltd. and OmniScriptum S.R.L publishing group

120 High Road, East Finchley, London, N2 9ED, United Kingdom
Str. Armeneasca 28/1, office 1, Chisinau MD-2012, Republic of Moldova, Europe
Printed at: see last page
ISBN: 978-620-7-30749-4

orthopaedics MCQS and clinical cases

Amel DJERBAL
Ahcene Said ouamer
Samir TEBANI

Table of Contents

Questions

Question 1:

A bite wound needs to be treated in a way that combines all these suggestions, except which one?

a- Primary wound suture
b- Debridement of the wound (trimming)
c- Complete cleansing and irrigation of the wound
d- Immobilisation of the wound
e- General antibiotic therapy with tetanus prevention

Question 2:

Galiazzi fracture, associated with a fracture of the radial diaphysis:

a- A fracture of the lower end of the radius
b- Dislocation of the radial head
c- A fracture of the olecranon
d- An inferior radiocubital dislocation
e- Dislocation of the elbow

Question 3:

One of these clinical signs of anteromedial dislocation of the shoulder is false.

a- Sign of the epaulette
b- Internal rotation of the arm
c- Vacuity of the glenoid
d- Filling of the delto-pectoral fold
e- Irreducible abduction

Question No 4:

All of the following statements about 1 child with acute osteomyelitis are correct, except one. Which is it?

a- Blood-borne infection of the bone
b- The germ most often responsible is staphylococcus aureus
c- It is generally located near the knee and far from the elbow
d- It is generally located in the diaphyseal region of the bone;
e- The radiograph is normal at the time of the first clinical signs

Question N°5 :

Complications of patella fractures are represented by :

1. The vicious callus
2. Stiff knees
3. Patellofemoral osteoarthritis
4. Instability of the knee

A : 1,3. B : 2,3,4 C : 1, 2, 3, 4 D: 1,2,4 E: 2,5

Question N° 6 :

The O'donoghue triad combines the following lesions:

1. External lateral ligament
2. Internal meniscus
3. Anterior cruciate ligament
4. Posterior cruciate ligament

A : 1, 2, 5 B : 1,3,4 C : 1, 2,3 D : 1,4,5 E : 2,4,5

Question N° 7 :

In articular fractures of the patella, mouley and richard type II corresponds to :

a. non-displaced transverse fracture
b. displaced transverse fracture
c. transverse fracture with cummunltlon of a fragment

d. community divide
e. sagittal fracture

Question N° 8 :

A trauma patient presents with a leg fracture. Clinical examination of the patient in bed shows that the kneecap is at its zenith, the outer edge of the foot is resting on the surface of the bed and the fractured leg is rotated. This attitude expresses :

a. angulation at the anterior vertex
b. an overlap
c. a time lag
d. a translation
e. angulation with a posterior apex

Question N° 9 :

The treatment of a transverse femoral neck fracture in a 35-year-old man is :

a. continuous traction
b. cervicocephalic arthroplasty
c. the pelvic-pedictic cast
d. reduction and osteosynthesis
e. total hip arthroplasty

Question N° 10 :

The treatment of a type I transverse open fracture of the middle third of the two leg bones, seen at the 3rd hour is :

a. the external fixator
b. centromedullary nailing
c. trans-calcanean traction
d. cruro-pedull plaster
e. screw-plate osteosynthesis

Question N° 11 :

The most characteristic complication of pertrochanteric fractures is :

a- Vicious callus

b- Pseudarthrosis
c- Necrosis of the femoral head
d- Coxarthrosis
e- Damage to the femoral artery

Question 12:

In the event of a fall from a high place, you should always look for the following injuries: (tick the wrong answer)

a- A spinal fracture
b- A fracture of the calcaneus
c- Fracture of the patella
d- A fracture of the tibial plateau
e- A fracture of the upper end of the femur

Question N° 13 :

Severe ankle sprains are characterised by :

a- Ligament distension
b- Capsulo-ligament distension
c- Total ligament rupture
d- Capsulo-ligament rupture
e- A rupture of the lateral peroneal tendon

Question N° 14 :

Osteosynthesis using a fixator is indicated in cases of :

a- Comminuted fracture
b- Fracture with significant displacement
c- Fracture with skin opening
d- Fracture with nerve damage
e- Non-displaced fracture

Question N° 15 :

One of these fracture displacements is poorly tolerated. Which is it?

a- Overlap
b- Anterior angulation
c- Internal time lag
d- External offset
e- Posterior apex angulation

Question N° 16 :

Treatment of an unstable fracture of the lumbar spine involves

a- Immobilisation with a plaster cast corset
b- Simple bed rest followed by rehabilitation
c- Osteosynthesis
d- Mobilisation and early rehabilitation
e- Bed traction

Question N° 17 :

Associated inversion of the foot: *(tick the wrong answer)*

a- Plantar flexion of the ankle
b- A varus foot
c- Adduction of the foot

d- Pronation of the foot
e- Internal rotation

Question N° 18 :

In true cervical fractures, there is communication:

a- In front of the femoral neck
b- Behind the femoral neck
c- In the cervical region
d- In the trochanteric region
e- In all these regions

Question N° 19 :

Identify the radiological signs in favour of an anteromedial shoulder of the subcoracoid variety on a frontal view:

2. humeral head under the coracoid
3. loss of sphericity of the humeral head
4. flattening of the glenoid
5. neck of the humerus projecting below the axillary edge of the scapula

A.1+2+5 B.1+2+4 C. 2+4+5 D.3+4+5 E. 1+3+5

Question N° 20 :

Of the following anatomical elements, only one is not a component of the Roy-Camille vertebral segment.

a. the posterior wall of the vertebral body
b. pedicles
c. the spinous process
d. isthmuses
e. the blades

Question N° 21 :

Which of the complications of fractures of the two bones of the forearm is the most serious and the most common?

a. injury to the median nerve
b. injury to the ulnar nerve
c. prono-supination stiffness
d. Wolkman syndrome
e. Radio-cubital synostosis

Question N° 22 :

Fat embolism may occur in the course of :

a- Long bone fractures
b- Dystocic delivery
c- Accidental intravenous injection of an oily substance
d- Open heart surgery
e- Accidental opening of the venous catheter under the keyboard.

Question N° 23 :

The treatment of open leg fractures type III (Cauchoix - Duparc) must include :

1. Surgical trimming of the soft tissue
2. Primary skin closure
3. Osteosynthesis of bone lesions using a screw plate
4. Immobilisation of bone injuries using an external fixator

A : 1, 2, 3 B : 1, 2, 4 C : 1, 2, 5 D : 1, 3, 5 E : 2, 3, 5

Question 24:

The BENNETT fracture is a fracture :

a. From the neck of the 5th metacarpal
b. From the neck of the 4th metacarpal
c. From the base of the 2nd metacarpal
d. Joint of the base of the 1st metacarpal bone
e. Extra-articular of the base of the 1st metacarpal

Question N° 25 :

The most common humeral palmar fracture in children is :

a- External condyle
b- Supra condyle
c- From the epitrochlea
d- From the epicondyle
e- The capitellum

Question N° 26 :

The treatment of a type II open leg fracture seen after the 6th hour is :

a. Screw-plate osteosynthesis
b. Osteosynthesis by centromedullary nailing
c. Osteosynthesis by external fixator
d. Cruro-pedious plaster
e. Plate blade osteosynthesis

Question N° 27 :

The average healing time for a single leg fracture is

a. 1 to 2 months
b. 7 to 8 months
c. 4 to 5 months
d. 8 to 12 months

e. More than 12 months

Question No 28 :

Loss of sensitivity of the shoulder stump in dislocation antero-medial shoulder evokes: (tick the right answer)

a. A vascular lesion
b. Musculocutaneous nerve damage
c. A vasculo-nerve lesion.
d. Involvement of the supraspinatus nerve
e. Circumflex nerve damage

Question No 29 :

Which of the following fractures of the humeral palette would result in a valgus ulna: (tick the right answer)

A. Of the medial condyle
B. Of the external condyle
C. From the epitrochlea
D. Dia-condylar
E. Sus and intercondylar

Question N° 30 :

In fractures of the upper end of the femur in elderly patients, mortality is linked to (tick the right answer)

A. The complexity of bone lesions
B. The association of vascular lesions
C. Disappointing surgical treatment
D. Decubitus complications
E. Necrosis of the femoral head

Question N° 31 :

On a 3A obturator X-ray of the pelvis, all but one of the following are visible. Which one: *(tick the right answer)*

a. the iliopubic line
b. the anterior column
c. the rear parol
d. the roof of the acetabulum
e. the ischio-pubic line

Question No 32 :

Which of the following traumatic dislocations of the hip do you think is the most common?

a. Anterior superior pubic
b. Antero inferior obturator
c. Posteroinferior Iliac
d. Posterior inferior ischiatic
e. All these proposals
f.

Question N° 33 :

In a polytrauma patient with a comminuted femur fracture, what are the signs in favour of fat embolism?

1. Atelectasis
2. throbopenia
3. Petechiae
4. hyperthermia

A: 1.2 B: 2.4 C: 2.3 D : 3.4 E: 1.4

Question No 34 :

A patient was admitted as an emergency with trauma to the lower leg. The neurological assessment revealed a loss of plantar flexion of the foot and toes and a reduction in supination and adduction.

You are talking about: *(tick the right answer)*

a. Injury to the external popliteal sciatic nerve
b. Injury to the medial popliteal sciatic nerve
c. Injury to the crural nerve
d. A lesion of the short saphenous nerve
e. Injury to the long saphenous nerve

Question N° 35 :

On monitoring a skull fracture with loss of consciousness, certain elements suggest an extra dural haematoma. Which one? *(tick the wrong answer)*

a. Worsening of consciousness after the first hour
b. Notion of a temporal fracture line
c. Immediately severe coma
d. Unilateral mydriasis
e. - Hemiplegia (delayed onset)

Question No 36 :

In a comatose polytrauma patient with a Glasgow Coma Scale score of 8, signs suggestive of cervical cord injury include: *(tick wrong answer)*

a. Areflexic and flaccid limbs
b. Diaphragmatic breathing
c. Fall in blood pressure with tachycardia
d. Priapism
e. Decreased anal sphincter tone

Question N° 37 :

Fractures of the humeral shaft in adults usually give rise to the following complications, except for one. Which one? *(tick the wrong answer)*

a. A vicious callus with diaphyseal overlap

b. Vicious angular callus
c. Pseudarthrosis
d. Radial nerve paralysis
e. Paralysis of the musculocutaneous nerve

Question N° 38 :

Fractures of the humeral shaft in adults usually give rise to the following complications, except for one. Which one? *(tick the wrong answer)*

a. The compression-extension mechanism
b. - Vicious angular callus
c. - Pseudarthrosis
d. Radial nerve paralysis
e. Paralysis of the musculocutaneous nerve

Question N° 39 :

Bimalleolar fractures treated orthopaedically are usually reduced by the . *(tick the right answer)*

a. Pilscher
b. Fevre
c. Maisonneuve
d. Boot puller
e. Supination of the foot

Question N° 40 :

Divergent elbow dislocation of the 2 bones of the forearm: (tick the right answer)

A- Determines dislocation anterior to the olecranon and posterior to the radial head

B- Determines dislocation behind the olecranon and in front of the radial head

C- Determines dislocation behind the two bones of the forearm

D- Determines dislocation in front of the 2 bones of the forearm

E- Is frequent in elbow trauma

Question No 41 :

In the case of multivertebral disease with an infectious appearance, the most likely diagnosis is : (tick the correct answer)

A- Spinal staphylococcal disease

B- Hodgkin's disease

C- Brucellosis

D- Leishmaniasis

E- Vertebral haemangioma

Question No 42 :

The sagital fracture of the patella is: *(tick the wrong answer)*

A- A joint fracture

B- A fracture that ruptures the extensor apparatus

C- Confused with a bipartite patella

D- Treated by simple plaster cast immobilisation

E- Sometimes treated with an equatorial cerclage

Question No 43 :

The PUscher reduction manoeuvre is shown in: *(tick the right answer)*

A- Epiphyseal detachment

B- Fracture of the radial head

C- Pouteau Colles' fracture

D- Goyrand Smith fracture

E- Fracture of the lower quarter of the radius

Question N° 44 :

In a Pouteau Colles fracture, all of the following displacements are found, except one. Which one? *(tick the correct answer)*

A- Ascension of the radial styloid
B-External translation
C- Metaphyseal impaction
D - Exaggerated anterior tilt
E- Horizontalisation of the frontal tilt

Question N° 45 :

A fracture of the neck of the femur classified as Pauwels III corresponds to : *(tick the right answer)*

A- A horizontal fracture
B- A vertical fracture
C- A fracture subjected to compressive forces
D- A fracture that usually consolidates well
E- No correct answer

Question No 46 :

The diagnosis of a traumatic anteromedial dislocation of the shoulder is made on the basis of: *(tick the right answer)*

A- Sign of the epaulette

B- Sign of the external axe strike
C- Irreducible adduction
D- Irreducible abduction
E. Circumflex nerve paralysis

Question No 47 :

One complication is particularly feared in the case of a fracture of the two bones of the adult forearm: *(tick the right answer)*

A- Radial paralysis
B- Ulnar paralysis
C- Stiffness in elbow flexion-extension
D- Stiffness of the prono-supinatlon
E- Algo-dystrophic syndrome

Question No 48 :

In the event of a dashboard syndrome, an injured person presents with flexion-adduction-internal rotation of the limb, the most likely diagnosis is: *(tick the right answer)*

A- A highly displaced femoral neck fracture
B- A trochanteric fracture
C- A fracture of the acetabulum
D- High coxofemoral dislocation
E- Low coxofemoral dislocation

Question 49:

You receive a patient who has suffered a trauma to the dorsolumbar spine with neurological damage. This paralysis will be assessed according to: *(tick the right answer)*

2. Sensory level
3. Engine level
4. The vegetative level
5. None of the above

A: 1,2,3 B: 2,3,4 C: 3,4,5 D: 1,3,5 E: 1,3, 4

Question N° 50 :

the level of paraplegia in a patient with anaesthesia from the umbilicus is: *(tick the right answer)*

A-D6
B-D7

C-D8
D-D9
E-D10

Clinical cases

Clinical case N°1

A 60-year-old patient with no previous history of any particular injury came to emergency with a traumatic injury to his right hand. When he fell on his hand, he felt pain and a cracking sensation; the functional importance was total and the patient presented supporting his right wrist with his valid hand.

You suspect a compression-extension fracture of the lower extremity of the radius.

What clinical signs are you looking for to confirm your diagnosis?

1. horizontalisation of the bistyoid line
2. external deviation of the hand
3. a fork-shaped deformity
4. a fork-bellied deformity
5. A drooping hand

1+2+3 B. 1+2+3... C. 1+2+4+5 D. 4+5 E. 1+2+4

What are the radiological signs?

A. A transverse metaphyseal line
B. Subsequent comminution
C. A rear gear
D. A posterior tilt
E. All these signs can bc found

This lesion can be found in all but one of these cases. Which is it?

A- Potential Castaing fracture
B- Poutteau Colles fracture
C- Gérard Marchand fracture
D- Associated carpal bone fracture
E - Goyrand Smith fracture

At this stage, treatment involves a number of principles.

1. Manual rehabilitation using traction flexion ulnar inclination
2. Stabilisation by pinning
3. Cast immobilisation
4. Initial osteosynthesis
5. Wrist rehabilitation

A: 1,2,3 B: 1,2,3,5 C:1,2,4 D: 1,4,5 E: 4,5

The secondary complications of this type of fracture are :

A- Secondary displacement
B- Instability of the carpus
C- Reflex algoneurodystrophy
D- Carpal tunnel syndrome
E- All these lesions are possible

Clinical case N°2

An 87-year-old man, retired in his own home and still gardening and walking alone to the market 500 metres from his home, fell from a height and was unable to get up. He was examined urgently and complained of acute pain in his right groin. He was carried in a stretcher by his neighbours, and on examination was found to have a soft, painful swelling in the groin and an externally rotated position of the right lower limb. Attempting to mobilise him caused severe pain.

The vicious attitude of the affected limb must then show the following clinical signs on inspection:

1. Internal rotation
2. Lengthening
3. Shortening
4. External rotation
5. Supply

A. 1+2+3...........B.2+3+4...........C.3+4+5 ....D.1+2+4...........E.2+3+5

The greatest risk to this elderly man, who is confined to bed, is :

A. Hip stiffness
B. Pseudarthrosis
C. A vital risk
D. Necrosis of the femoral head
E. The vicious callus

The principle treatment for this 87-year-old man who is still able to walk is :

A- Therapeutic abstention
B- Simple bed rest
C- Surgical treatment
D- Immobilisation in a pelvic-pedictic cast
E- Early rehabilitation with physiotherapy

The most appropriate treatment is therefore :

A- Traction suspension using a transtibial pin
B- Synthesis of the fracture
C- Placement of a cervicocephalic prosthesis
D- Placement of a cup on the femoral head
E- Cervico-cephalic endouage

Clinical case N°3

A young judoka, aged 24, was admitted to emergency following a fall to the ground, with his right upper limb in abduction and external rotation. Examination showed an obvious "DES- SAULT" attitude, with adduction of the arm impossible on the right.

Clinical examination reveals all these signs, except one. Which is it? (tick the wrong answer)

A- Filling of the deltopectoral groove
B- Abduction impossible.
C- External axe strike
D- The epaulette sign
E- Vacuity of the glenoid

Normally, the radiological work-up to be requested should include: (tick the right answer)

1. Front X-ray
2. Axillary profile X-ray
3. Trans-thoracic profile radiograph
4. Incidence of LAMY
5. Incidence of BERNAGEAU

A: 1.5 B: 1.3 C:2.5 , D:2.4 E: 1.4

What is your emergency treatment approach? (tick the right answer)

1. Reduction under general anaesthetic
2. Open-cast reduction
3. 21-day restraint
4. 10-day restraint
5. Rehabilitation from the outset

A: 1.4 B: 2.3 , C : 1.5 D: 1.3 E: 2.4

Of the following complications, the most frequently encountered is:
(tick the right answer)

A- Necrosis of the humeral head
B- Retractable capsule
C- Brachial plexus paralysis
D- Recurrence
E- Vicious callus of the upper end of the humeral head

Clinical case N°4

Mrs A. Baya, aged 70, fell from a height onto her right side. She experienced severe pain and was unable to get up. Her functional impotence was total and the pain was exacerbated by any attempt to mobilise her. X-rays of the pelvis showed a true trans-cervical fracture displaced in coxa vara, with the cephalic bone trabeculae oblique in prolongation but offset.

Your practical attitude will consist of: (tick the right answer)

1. Detecting shock
2. Look for associated trauma
3. Look for vascular and nerve complications
4. Look for associated clinical defects
5. Temporary immobilisation and radiography

A: 1,2,3,5 B: 3,4,5 C: 1,3,5, D: 2,4,5 E: 1,2

Of these additional tests, only one is unusual. Which one?

A- Front X-ray, right hip in internal rotation
B- Front chest X-ray
C- Front radiograph of right hip in external rotation
D- Complete pre-operative biological work-up with ECG
E- X-ray of the spine if spinal anaesthesia is planned

According to GARDEN, this lesion is of the following type: (tick the right answer)

A. I
B. II
C. III
D. IV
E. Unclassifiable

In this field and in front of this painting, your treatment will be: **(tick**

the right answer)

A- Cervico-cephalic reduction and osteosynthesis
B- External fixer
C- Continuous extension
D- Cervico-cephalic prosthesis
E- Abstentions and seating

Clinical case N°5 :

A young footballer suffers a sports accident in a tackle. He was hit by his opponent's foot on the anterointebral side of his right leg where the middle 1/3 and lower 1/3 meet. He immediately developed total functional impotence with severe leg pain.
There is an immediate deformity of the leg with an anterointebral crook.
In addition, there was a 4 cm linear cut with irregular, contused edges from which blood mixed with droplets of fat was coming out.

It is therefore a: (tick the right answer)

A- Fracture of 2 leg bones
B- Open fracture
C- Soft tissue wound
D- Joint wound
E- Fracture complicated by vascular lesion

X-rays normally show displacement, especially in : (tick the right answer)

A. Offset
B. Pure overlap
C. Shortening
D. Angulation
E. Compression

The emergency treatment consists of : *(tick the right answer)*

1. Antibiotic therapy
2. Tetanus serotherapy
3. External mounting
4. Plaster cast
5. Continuous traction

A: 1, 2,5 B: 1,2 C: 3, D: 1,2,3 E: 1,5

After surgical trimming, the wound was able to be closed with the skin stretched taut. It is a skin lesion of the following type: *(tick the right answer)*

A- I by Cauchoix and Duparc
B- He of Cauchoix and Duparc
C- III by Cauchoix and Duparc
D- IV de Mechelany
E- V by Mechelanv

Clinical case N°6 :

A 25-year-old patient was admitted in an emergency with the following clinical presentation: state of traumatic shock, total functional impotence and pain in the right lower limb, flexion adduction internal rotation deformity of the same limb.

In this patient, the clinical deformity immediately suggests: *(tick the right answer)*

A- A hip fracture
B- A trochantero-cervical fracture
C- Anterior dislocation of the hip variety
D- A dislocated hip fracture of the posterior variety
E- Posterior dislocation of the hip isolated or associated with a fracture

The emergency radiology work-up for this patient includes these views: *(tick the wrong answer)*

A- Face of the "débrouillage" basin
B- Three-quarter length
C- Three-quarter shutter
D- Profile of the hip
E- External rotation of the foot

There was pain in the abdomen and buttocks. X-rays of the front and side reveal a dislocation of the hip and a fracture of the hip bone. The clinical examination should focus on a common complication, which one?

A. Sciatic paralysis
B. A femoral paralysis
C. Femoral thrombosis
D. A posterior skin opening
E. A haematoma on the buttock

The first treatment for bone lesions is: *(tick the right answer)*

A. Reduction of the dislocation
B. Osteosynthesis of the acetabulum
C. Continued expansion
D. The fitting of a hip prosthesis
E. Cast immobilisation.

In all these cases, surgery is indicated from the outset: *(tick the wrong answer)*

A- Intra-articular incarceration of a bone fragment
B- Irreducibility
C- Associated femoral head fracture
D- Vascular lesions
E- Involvement of the lateral popliteal sciatica

The most common long-term complications are: *(tick the right answer)*

1. Osteonecrosis of the femoral head
2. Pseudarthrosis of the femoral neck
3. Coxartfirose
4. Ankylosis of the hip
5. Recurrent hip dislocation

A: 1.2 B: 1.3 C: 1.4 D : 4.5 E: 3.5

Clinical case N°7

A 55-year-old woman fell on the palm of her hand with her wrist in extension. She presented to emergency with a large, painful and deformed wrist. From the front, there was an external shift of the hand; from the side, there was a posterior distal deformity of the wrist and dorsal recoil of the hand.

Radiological analysis concluded that the fracture was a Pouteau Colles fracture. One of these architectural changes is not correct. Which one? (tick the correct answer)

- A- Horizontalization of the bi-styloid line
- B- Ulnar styloid fracture
- C- Shortening of the radius
- D- Radial glenoid looking down and back
- E- Inversion of the inferior radio-ulnar index finger

What complication may accompany this fracture? *(tick the right answer)*

- A- A punctiform skin opening at the ulnar edge of the wrist
- B- Algodystrophic syndrome
- C- Secondary displacement after orthopaedic treatment
- D- Comminution of the posterior cortex
- E- All these answers are correct

The reduction criteria for this fracture to be looked for on the frontal and lateral views are: *(tick the wrong answer)*

- A. Restoring the bi-styloid line
- B. Restoring the lower radio-ulnar index
- C. Recovery of normal radius length
- D. Orientation of the radial glenoid downwards and forwards on the profile
- E. Crossing the posterior cortex

Treatment of the fracture will preferably involve : *(tick the right answer)*

A- A cast for 6 weeks
B- Kapandji type intra-focal pinning
C- Bloody reduction and Py-type pinning
D- Orthopaedic reduction and external fixator
E- Bloody reduction and external fixator.

Clinical case N°8

A 24-year-old driver, the victim of a collision, was admitted to a specialist hospital in an emergency the same day.

The clinical examination on admission showed an immediate onset of coma with a Glasgow Coma Scale score of 8, a haemorrhagic wound on the right temporal scalp, polypnoea at 30/min with cyanosis of the extremities and sweating, a heart rate of 110/min, a blood pressure of 80/60 mm Hg, and an anterolateral lac of the right thigh.

All these diagnostic hypotheses are possible, except one. Which is it?

A- Extra-dural haematoma
B- Haemothorax
C- Femur fracture
D- Haemoperitoneum
E- Pulmonary contusion

The emergency biological assessment must include the following tests:

1. Blood count
2. Liver transaminases
3. Sedimentation rate
4. Blood grime
5. Grouping

A: 1,2,3 B: 1,2,4 C: 1,4,5 D: 1,3,5 E: 3,4,5

All of these emergency radiological investigations are useful for diagnosis, except one. Which is it?

A- X-rays of the skull, front and side
B- Chest X-ray
C- Radiography of the femur
D- Cerebral tomography
E- Abdominal ultrasound

The secondary radiological work-up will be completed by all these investigations, except one. Which is it?

A- Radiography of the pelvis
B- Radiography of the spine
C- X-ray of the knee
D- Unprepared abdominal X-ray
E- Costal grill

Which of these clinical and biological factors gives the best indication of the severity of an acute haemorrhagic anaemia?

A- Pallor
B- Blood pressure level
C- Haemoglobin level
D- Haematocrit rate
E- Red blood cell count

While waiting for a blood transfusion, all these filling solutions can be used, except one. Which is it?

A- 0.9% isotonic saline solution
B- 5% isotonic glucose serum + electrolytes
C- Plasmagel
D- 10% Mannitol
E- Fresh frozen plasma (FFP)

After filling: partial correction of shock but worsening of signs of respiratory distress and appearance of venous hyperpressure (turgidity of the jugular veins).
Among the diagnostic hypotheses. Which is false?

A- Suffocating pleural effusion
B- Suffocating haemomediastinum
C- Hemopericardium
D- Haemoperitoneum
E- Pulmonary contusion

The chest X-ray showed posterolateral fractures of the 3rd, 4th and 6th right ribs and a poorly defined opaque parenchymatous image of the right middle and upper lobes. The parenchymal lesion is related to :

A- Right atelectasis
B- Right intrapulmonary haematoma
C- Inhalation-induced pulmonary oedema
D- Right pulmonary contusion
E- Cardiogenic oedema due to overload

What treatment should be given for these parenchymal and fracture lesions?

A. Artificial ventilation alone
B. Osteosynthesis of the fracture site
C. A + B
D. Artificial ventilation + thoracic analgesia
E. No proposal

In an emergency situation and after controlling circulatory and respiratory distress, what treatment should be given for encephalitis?

A. Surgical treatment alone
B. Cerebral edema treatment alone
C. A + B
D. Puncture of the 4th ventricle + external drainage
E. Ventriculoperitoneal bypass

Neurological resuscitation treatment will include all these elements, except one. Which is it?

A- Mannitol 10% infusion
B- Intravenous (IV) corticosteroids
C- Artificial ventilation
D- IV vasodilators
E- IV glycerol

Which of the following complications may arise in the immediate aftermath and require emergency fixation of the right femoral shaft fracture site?

A- Pulmonary embolism
B- Opening the fracture site
C- Muscle tear
D- Fat embolism
E- Compression of the sciatic nerve

Clinical case N°9 :

A.A, aged 32, was admitted to the trauma department in a state of shock following a road traffic accident.
Emergency examination reveals

- A point of impact on the right thorax and lower limbs.
- A soiled open fracture of the lower 1/4 of the left leg with loss of substance.
- A fracture of the right humeral shaft with loss of flexion and extension of the fingers and wrist, and anaesthesia of the thenar and 3 outer fingers.

Within half an hour of arrival, the patient presents with hypovolaemic shock. The most reliable factor is?

A- Anemia
B- Low or even impregnable blood pressure
C- Very low central venous pressure
D- Tachycardia
E- Cyanosis

On discharge from intensive care, the patient was seen at the 12th hour by the orthopaedic surgeon, who decided on an open fracture:

A- Local antibiotic therapy
B- General antibiotic therapy
C- Surgical trimming
D- Cast immobilisation
E- Low-dose corticosteroid therapy

To complete the medical procedure, it is essential to do the following:

A- Suturing with drainage
B- Suturing without drainage
C- To perform an amputation
D- To leave open

E- To make a simple skin approximation

On day 3, this fracture was labelled a type II open leg fracture. The treatment of choice will consist of :

A- Transcalcaneal traction
B- A cruro-pedious plaster cast
C- A centromedullary endouage
D- An external fixator
E- Amputation

On day 6, the left foot was cold and insensitive, with necrosis of the toes and no pedal pulse. The decision was made to amputate:

A- Whose seat is at the bottom 1/3
B- Whose seat is in the top 1/4
C- Whose seat is at the top 1/3
D- Whose seat is 1/4 lower
E- Where the seat is in the middle 1/3

This amputation, carried out at an ideal level using the osteo-myoplastic technique, will make all these suggestions possible, except one. And that is?

A- A classic socket
B- Equal distribution of pressure
C- A "contact" fitting
D- Concervation of the trophidity of the stump
E- Active restraint

Nerve damage in the upper limb should be investigated:

A- Injury to the median nerve alone
B- Injury to the median and ulnar nerves
C- Damage to the radial nerve
D- Injury to the median and radial nerves
E- Damage to 3 nerves

At 6 months, the wrist and finger extensors had recovered. There is still a sensory-motor deficit in the thumb, opposition and wrist flexion.

This is a :

A- Radial axonotmesis and medial neurapraxia
B- Ulnar axonotmesis and radial neurapraxia
C- Median neurotmesis and ulnar axonotmesis
D- Median neurotmesis and radial neurapraxia
E- Radial neurotmesis and ulnar neurapraxia

Reviewed at the 12th month, the loss of opposition was bothering the patient. A re-intervention was decided. All these factors are essential for success, except one. Which is it?

A - Flexible finger joints
B- A transferable muscle on side 4
C- Persistence of anaesthesia in the outer fingers
D- A transferable muscle with an interferenbel pattern
E- A transferable muscle with a rich intermediate trace

Clinical case N°10

Mr A.B, aged 50, a non-insulin-dependent diabetic, was hit by a vehicle that day. He was evacuated to emergency with the following clinical picture: sweating, agitation, obnubilation, polypnoea, BP 70/50mmHg, pulse 125/mn, right lower limb deformity with skin opening.

Clinical examination revealed abdominal guarding with ecchymosis at the base of the right thorax and an impaction filling the homolateral lumbar fossa. Pulmonary auscultation shows an abolition of the right vesicular murmur with dullness of the base: (tick the wrong answer)

A- Renal contusion
B- Hepatic trauma
C- Haemothorax
D- Peritonitis
E- Subperitoneal bladder rupture

At this stage, a number of investigations are necessary for diagnosis, except one. Which is it?

A- Abdominal scan
B- Renal arteriography
C- Renal ultrasound
D- Peritoneal lavage puncture
E- Intravenous urography

Management of this patient's life-threatening condition requires all but one of the following procedures. Which is it?

A- Vascular filling
B- Venous approaches
C- Artificial ventilation
D- Freeing the airways
E- Oxygen therapy via nasal tube

Blood glucose (with dextrostix) is above 2.5gr/l.

Pending confirmation by the laboratory, you should administer :

A- Hypoglycaemic sulphonamides

B- Mannitol

C- Glucose serum

D- Insulin delay

E- Ordinary insulin

X-ray examination shows a horizontal linear fracture of the right leg. Your immediate response will be :

A- Classify this fracture according to the Cauchoix and Duparc classification.

B- Immobilise the limb with a cruropedic cast

C- Apply a flat dressing and stabilise immediately with a cast

D- Perform surgical trimming and place the patient under continuous extension

E- Perform surgical trimming and stabilise the focus as a matter of urgency

The chest X-ray shows the following lesion:

A- Round opacity

B- Hemithoracic hyperclarity

C- Right atelectasis

D- Meniscal opacity

E- An accentuation of the vascular network

During the course of the discasc, the patient presented with a systolic BP of 70 mm Hg, tachycardia, a very low PVC and oligoanuria. These are:

A- Cardiogenic shock

B- Hypovolaemic shock

C- Septic shock

D- Pericarditis j|

E- Pulmonary embolism

What treatment would you suggest in this situation?

A- Digoxin IV

B- Isoprenaline infusion
C- IV corticosteroid therapy
D- Lasilix IV
E- Perfusion of macromolecules

Intraoperative examination revealed haemoperitoneum, a linear liver wound, a non-pulsatile right retroperitoneal haematoma and a diaphragmatic breach.

What should I do?

2. Suture of the liver wound and diaphragmatic rupture
3. Evacuation and drainage of hemoperitoneum
4. Chest drainage
5. Respect for retroperitoneal haematoma

A: 1,2,3,4 B:1,2,4,5 C: 1,3,4,5 D: 2,3 E: 1,2,3,5

Answers
Questions

Question 1:

a- Primary wound suture

Question 2:

d- An inferior radiocubital dislocation

Question 3:

b- Internal rotation of the arm

Question No 4:

d- It is generally located in the diaphyseal region of the bone.

Question 5

C: 1, 2, 3, 4

Question N° 6 :

B : 1, 3, 4

Question N° 7 :

c- transverse fracture with accumulation of a fragment

Question N° 8 :

c- a time lag

Question N° 9 :

d- reduction and osteosynthesis

Question N° 10 :

b- centromedullary nailing

Question N° 11 :

a- Vicious callus

Question 12:

c- Fracture of the patella

Question N° 13 :

b- Capsulo-ligament rupture

Question N° 14 :

c- Fracture with skin opening

Question N° 15 :

c- Internal time lag

Question N° 16 :

c- Osteosynthesis

Question N° 17 :

d- Pronation of the foot

Question N° 18 :

b- Behind the femoral neck

Question N° 19 :

A.1+2+5

Question N° 20 :

c- spinous process

Question N° 21 :

d- Wolkman syndrome

Question N° 22 :

a- Long bone fractures

Question N° 23 :

C : 1,2,5

Question 24:

d- Joint at the base of the 1st metacarpal bone

Question N° 25 :

b- Supra condyle

Question N° 26 :

c- Osteosynthesis by external fixator

Question N° 27 :

c- 4 to 5 months

Question No 28 :

e- Circumflex nerve damage

Question No 29 :

B- External condyle

Question N° 30 :

D- Decubitus complications

Question N° 31 :

a. the ischio-pubic line

Question No 32 :

c- Posteroinferior Iliac

Question N° 33 :

D : 3,4

Question No 34 :

b- Injury to the medial popliteal sciatic nerve

Question N° 35 :

c- Immediately severe coma

Question No 36 :

b- Diaphragmatic breathing

Question N° 37 :

e- Musculocutaneous nerve paralysis

Question N° 38 :

d- Radial nerve paralysis

Question N° 39 :

d- Boot puller

Question N° 40 :

B- Determines dislocation behind the olecranon and in front of the radial head

Question No 41 :

A- Spinal staphylococcal disease

Question No 42 :

B A fracture that ruptures the extensor apparatus

Question No 43 :

C- Pouteau Colles' fracture

Question N° 44 :

D - Exaggerated anterior tilt

Question N° 45 :

B- A vertical fracture

Question No 46 :

C- Irreducible adduction

Question No 47 :

D- Stiffness of the prono-supinatlon

Question No 48 :

E- Low coxo-femoral dislocation Question N° 49 :

A: 1, 2, 3

Question N° 50 :

E- D10

Answers
Clinical cases

Clinical case N°1

1+2+3

A- All these signs can be found

E- Goyrand Smith fracture

A : 1, 2,3

E- All these lesions are possible

Clinical case N°2

C. 3+4+5

A- A vital risk

C- Surgical treatment

C- Placement of a cervicocephalic prosthesis

Clinical case N°3

B- Abduction impossible.

B : 1,3

D: 1,3

D- Recurrence

Clinical case N°4

E: 1,2

C- Front radiograph of right hip in external rotation

D. IV

D- Cervico-cephalic prosthesis

Clinical case N°5 :

B- Open fracture

A- Angulation

D : 1, 2, 3

B- He of Cauchoix and Duparc

Clinical case N°6 :

E- Posterior dislocation of the hip isolated or associated with a fracture

External rotation of the foot

A- Sciatic paralysis

A- Reduction of the dislocation

E- Involvement of the lateral popliteal sciatica

B : 1,3

Clinical case N°7

B- Ulnar styloid fracture

E- All these answers are correct

A- Crossing the posterior cortex

B- Kapandji type intra-focal pinning

Clinical case N°8

A- Extra-dural haematoma C: 1, 4, 5

A- X-rays of the skull, front and side

D- Unprepared abdominal X-ray

B- Blood pressure level

D- 10% Mannitol

D- Haemoperitoneum

Right pulmonary contusion

Artificial ventilation + thoracic analgesia

A- Treatment for cerebral edema alone

D- IV vasodilators

D- Fat embolism

Clinical case N°9

C- Very low central venous pressure

C- Surgical trimming

E- To make a simple skin approximation

D- An external fixator

E- Where the seat is in the middle 1/3

A- A classic socket

D- Injury to the median and radial nerves

D- Median neurotmesis and radial neurapraxia

C- Persistence of anaesthesia in the outer fingers

Clinical case N°10

E- Subperitoneal bladder rupture

B- Renal arteriography

C- Artificial ventilation

E- Ordinary insulin

A- Classify this fracture according to the Cauchoix classification
and Duparc

D- Meniscal opacity

B- Hypovolaemic shock

E- Perfusion of macromolecules

D : 2,3

References

01. Resnick D: Radiology of the talocalcaneal joint. Radiology 111: 581-586, 1974.
02. Mann RA: Biomechanics of the foot. Instruct Course Lect 31: 167 180, 1982.
03. Kitaoka HB, Alexander IJ, Adelaar RS, et al. Clinical rating system; for the ankle-hindfoot, midfoot, hallux, and lesser toes. Foo! Ankle Int.15 : 349-353,1994.
04. Conway and J.J. Cowell HR: Tarsal coalition: clinical significance anc roentgenographic demonstration. Radiology 92(4): 799-809 1969.
05. Lateur LM, Van Hoe LR,Van Ghillewe KV, SS Gryspeerdt Baert AL Dereymaeker GE (1994). Subtalar coalition: diagnosis with the (sign on lateral radiographs of the ankle. Radiology193 (3) : 847 51.
06. Herzenberg JE, Goldner JL, Martinez S, Silverman PM Computerized tomography of talocalcaneal tarsal coalition: i clinical and anatomic study. Foot Ankle 6(6): 273--288, 1986.
07. Pineda C, Resnick D, Greenway G: Diagnosis of tarsal coalition with computed tomography. Clin Orthop Relat Res 208: 282 - 288, 1986.
08. Wilde PH, Torode IP, Dickens DR, Cole WG: Resection of symptomatic talocalcaneal coalition. J Bone Joint Surg Br 76(5) 797-801, 1994.
09. Rozansky A,Varley E , Moor M, Wenger DR, Mubarak SJ ; A radiologic classification of talocalcaneal coalition based on 3D reconstruction. J Child Orthop. Apr ; 4(2) : 129--35, 2010.
10. Kernbach KJ, DPM, Barkan H, Dr PH, Blitz NM; A Critical Evaluation Of Subtalar Joint Arthrosis Associated With Middle Facet Talocalcaneal Coalition in 21 Surgically Managed Patient A Retrospective Computed Tomography Review. Investigation; Involving Middle Facet Coalitions-Part III. clin Podiatr Med Surç 27, 135--143, 2010.

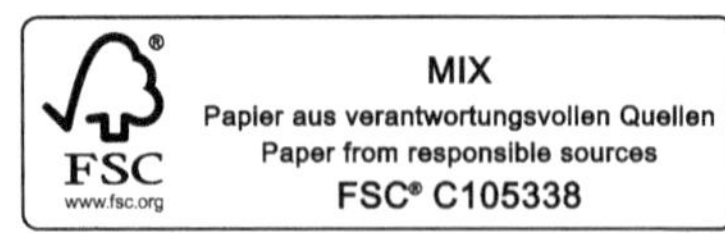

Printed by Books on Demand GmbH, Norderstedt / Germany